A Fountain of Gardens

21 Effective Galactagogues to Promote Lactation, Enrich Breast Milk Supply, and Improve Let-Down

Jennifer Elisabeth Maiden

Vintage Rose Natural Nursing
https://www.lovingmilkmaid.com

Bountiful Fruits:
https://www.bountifulfruits.com

CONTENTS

A Brief Introduction

For generations, many women have practiced the art of inducing non-maternal lactation for a variety of reasons, often discovering that they were able to produce sufficient quantities of healthy, nutrient-enriched breast milk even without nature's finest aids of pregnancy and childbirth. It is simply in a woman's nature to produce milk as a means of sustenance and nourishment, and very little can hinder her ability to do so. Over the years, women who have never experienced biological motherhood, those who have undergone hysterectomies, and even some who are post-menopausal have found success--and great pleasure-- in the journey of lactation.

The process of producing non-maternal lactation is not an easy one; as a matter of fact, it is a true labor of love, one that takes a great deal of concentrated effort, persistence and determination, and a lot of old-fashioned hard work that involves a very regulated schedule of proper breast stimulation, which can be achieved through suckling, manual expression, breast pump stimulation, and even the use of a TENS unit. Although this may seem rather daunting, women who truly desire lactation should not be discouraged; the goal of making breast milk *can* be achieved. It's just very important to take an honest and realistic approach to the process of lactation.

Lactation occurs in ten levels, and three stages known as Lactogenesis. The first of these three stages relies strictly upon proper hormone placement to ensure successful lactation, a process that occurs naturally during pregnancy. When inducing lactation, or encouraging the re-lactation process without the aid of pregnancy, these hormones must be set into place using alternative methods. Because the brain, body, and breasts must work together and believe that there is a need to produce breast milk, women will often encourage the process along with the use of lactogenic foods and herbs, also referred to as galactagogues.

Within her garden of gold, Mother Nature provides wonderful sources of chlorophyll, phytoestrogens, vitamins, minerals, and nutrients essential to the lactation process in the form of fruits, vegetables, plants, and herbs, and while many of these estrogenic herbs regulate important internal hormone levels, making them very effective in the pursuit of building breast milk, they are not typically meant for long-term use. Instead, they are added into a daily lactation routine as a means of kick-starting the milk-making process and helping to build a supply that a woman will then manage and maintain on her own, through suckling and proper milk removal, which occurs during the third and final stage of Lactogenesis. Long-term use of fresh and healthy lactogenic super foods is a better choice, as eating a well-balanced diet for good health and longevity is important for every woman--whether she is lactating or not.

Galactagogues can also be an effective method of increasing, supporting, and enriching an already established supply of milk, and are often used to aid breastfeeding mothers who suffer from chronic low milk supply, or adoptive mothers who long to nourish and nurture their new bundles of joy.

As a nursing woman who was blessed to breastfeed three children, I understand the importance and value of lactation and producing plentiful quantities of nutritious breast milk in order to nurture, nourish, and sustain the body and spirit. I wish you great success as you begin your beautiful journey into lactation and fulfill the dream of making a fountain of lovely liquid gold.

Jennifer Elisabeth Maiden
The Loving Milk Maid

A garden inclosed is *my sister,* my *spouse; a spring shut up, a fountain sealed.*

Thy plants are *an orchard of pomegranates, with pleasant fruits; camphire with spikenard,*

Spikenard and saffron; calamus and cinnamon, with all trees of frankincense, myrrh and aloes, with all the chief spices:

A fountain of gardens, a well of living waters, and streams from Lebanon.

Song of Solomon, 4:12-15

Chapter 1
The Use of Galactagogues

A galactogogue, or lactogenic, is a herb or other substance, such as a prescription medication, that is used to help increase breast milk supply, and even improve the Milk Ejection Reflex (MER), or let-down reflex, in nursing women, and the decision to add herbal supplements into your daily lactation routine is a very personal one. For some women, herbs are a feasible option when hoping to encourage a swifter increase in breast milk supply, and, after a bit of deliberation, others may decide that herbs are not really right for them. There is currently a lactation product on the market that proclaims to be a "miracle in a bottle", which is quite misleading to women who long to lactate, or are suffering from chronic low milk supply. While it would be wonderful to have access to such a product, there is simply no miraculous or magical means of making more breast milk, and herbal supplements hold very stark realities. While they can aid in the lactation process, they will not simply make milk for you. Herbs and other lactogenic food sources simply help the process along, and taking them will require you to continue the use of applicable lactation techniques, such as suckling, hand expression, pumping, and/or TENS stimulation, and some women find that these methods remain more effective than taking supplements.

That is not to say that there is no success to be found from including lactogenic herbs (and nature's other finest super foods, which I myself use with fantastic results) in your lactation routine. There *is,* and many women have achieved wonderful results from the incorporation of herbs. Opinions and results vary greatly, of course, and it's very important to remember that not every woman will respond to herbal supplements in the same way, or in the same length of time.

Before we explore the most effective, and often commonly used, galactogogues, let's discuss what is already known about every herb.

- ❖ Herbs may be carefully packaged and stamped as "organically certified", but they are not FDA approved or regulated, and while they may have been prepared in a FDA-registered facility, this does not mean that they are FDA-certified.

- ❖ Even though they are natural, herbs should be used with caution, as you can suffer allergic reactions upon consumption, and even "overdose" if they are not consumed properly.

- ❖ Herbs do have side effect warnings.

- ❖ Herbs can negatively affect prescription medications, as they do carry drug interaction warnings with them.

- ❖ Some herbs are not recommended for women who are pregnant or currently nursing an infant.

- ❖ Herbal supplements can pass through breast milk, which means that your baby or partner will be taking them, too.

❖ It is important that you always check with a health care professional prior to beginning any herbal regimen.

The FDA does play some role in the production, marketing, and sale of all herbs, but they handle them as a food rather than as a medication, so their medicinal effectiveness is not proven or guaranteed to consumers.

While "fresh is usually best", when it comes to choosing an herbal galactagogue, it is better to opt for a dried root, leaf, flower, or seed, particularly if you will be using them as a tea or infusion. The process of drying fresh herbs locks in their medicinal, nutritive, and lactogenic properties, which leads to their effectiveness as galactagogues.

If you have been taking an herbal galactagogue for several weeks without achieving noticeable results in your milk supply, you might want to check your supplement for freshness. Dried herbs have very good color and distinct aromas. If the color of your herb seems dull or "faded", or has lost a lot of its color and aroma, it is probably old, and old herbs lose their effectiveness. Try replacing it with a new supply, and see if you notice an improvement.

Over time, and with repeated use, our bodies begin to adapt to new routines, and naturally build a tolerance for, or even a resistance to, certain medications; herbal supplements are no exception to this, and may attribute to a particular galactagogue's seemingly ineffective properties. If you have been using a lactogenic herb for several weeks without noticing results, your body may have built up an immunity to it. Try switching to a different lactogenic source, or combining a variety of galactagogues, to see if this helps.

Storing dried herbs in a glass airtight container with a well-fitting lid is the best way to preserve freshness, flavor, and nutritive properties. Placing them in a cool, dark, dry place will keep them fresh for a minimum of 18 months.

Please note that the herbs listed on the following pages of this guide are often used to aid in many health issues (ranging from diabetes and heart disease to digestive problems and kidney disorders), so I will not be focusing solely on their lactation properties, and because there are drug interaction warnings associated with these herbs, and the list is fairly extensive and not all-inclusive, I have used terms such as "some" and "several" as a generalization; you will need to check with your physician to ensure that a particular herb is right for you. If you are currently taking a prescription medication that is not listed beneath each medication interaction heading, it is recommended that you speak with a qualified health care professional to be sure that combining your medication with a galactagogue is safe for you. Although some herbs are commonly listed here, and in other herbal resources, as safe for pregnant women, always use your own judgment when taking any herbal supplement, as many are estrogenic and highly hormonal, and may be unsafe, particularly if you are at a risk for miscarriage.

Chapter 2
21 Effective Galactagogues

Alfalfa
(Medicago sativa)

❖ Alfalfa is a perennial flowering plant in the pea family.

❖ Alfalfa is commonly known as *lucerne* in the United Kingdom, South Africa, Australia, and New Zealand.

❖ Alfalfa is said to promote the development of the glandular tissue of the breasts. It increases both milk supply and the fat content of breast milk, and is traditionally prescribed to promote the function of the pituitary gland, the source of the main hormones for lactation, making it a great choice for increasing breast milk production.

❖ Alfalfa is highly nutritious, easy to absorb, and rich in chlorophyll, a host of minerals, such as calcium, magnesium, phosphorus, potassium, silicon, and zinc, and vitamins A, B1, B2, B3, B5, B6, C, D, E, and K, as well as essential and non-essential amino acids.

❖ Alfalfa is thought to lower total cholesterol and "bad" low-density lipoprotein (LDL) cholesterol.

Although an estrogenic herb that can be taken to promote menstruation, alfalfa is thought to be relatively safe when taken during pregnancy. However, be sure not to exceed the maximum recommended dosage, and to be certain that alfalfa is a safe choice for you, consult your doctor before taking it.

Alfalfa is safe for most adults, but taking it for an extended period of time or in a dose larger than what is suggested is not recommended, as it can cause symptoms that are similar to the autoimmune disease lupus.

As a non-lactogenic medicinal, Alfalfa is often used to treat or prevent the following conditions and illnesses:

- ❖ Kidney problems
- ❖ Bladder problems
- ❖ Prostate problems
- ❖ Asthma
- ❖ Arthritis
- ❖ Diabetes
- ❖ Upset stomach

Precautions to consider before taking Alfalfa:

- ❖ Decrease or discontinue use if you detect an oversupply of breast milk.
- ❖ Alfalfa may lower the effectiveness of the medication Warfarin.

Alfalfa may cause an allergic reaction in people who are allergic to:

- Peanuts
- Legumes

Use precaution when taking Alfalfa if you are currently being treated for the following disorders:

- Blood disorders

Alfalfa may cause the following side effects:

- Sensitivity to sunlight
- Sunburn
- Skin blistering
- Skin rash

Speak to your doctor before taking Alfalfa if you are currently taking the following over the counter or prescription medications:

- Azathioprine
- Basiliximab
- Cyclosporine
- Daclizumab
- muromonab-CD3
- Orthoclone
- Mycophenolate
- Tacrolimus
- Sirolimus
- Prednisone
- Corticosteroids
- Ciprofloxacin
- Lomefloxacin

- ❖ Ofloxacin
- ❖ Levofloxacin
- ❖ Sparfloxacin
- ❖ Gatifloxacin
- ❖ Moxifloxacin
- ❖ Trimethoprim/sulfamethoxazole
- ❖ Tetracycline
- ❖ Methoxsalen
- ❖ Trioxsalen
- ❖ Some birth control pills
- ❖ Estrogen pills

Anise
(Pimpinella anisum)

- ❖ Anise is also known as *aniseed*.
- ❖ Because of its black licorice flavor, anise is often used in Western cuisine as a flavoring for food, beverages, and candies.
- ❖ Anise is used to bring about lactation and alleviate menstrual discomfort.
- ❖ It is also thought to be an aphrodisiac.
- ❖ In general, Anise is considered safe when taken by healthy adults.

Anise is listed as **unsafe** during pregnancy. Because it has been used in traditional medicine to promote menstruation, it is believed that anise could trigger miscarriage. **Do not** use anise while pregnant.

As a non-lactogenic medicinal, Anise is often used to treat or prevent the following illnesses:

- ❖ Asthma

- ❖ Certain sleep disorders
- ❖ Cough
- ❖ Psoriasis

Precautions to consider before taking Anise:

- ❖ **Do not** confuse Anise with Japanese star anise, which is **toxic.**

Anise may cause an allergic reaction in people who are allergic to:

- ❖ Asparagus
- ❖ Caraway
- ❖ Celery
- ❖ Coriander
- ❖ Cumin
- ❖ Dill
- ❖ Fennel

Use precaution when taking Anise if you are currently being treated for the following disorders:

- ❖ Breast cancer
- ❖ Uterine cancer
- ❖ Ovarian cancer
- ❖ Endometriosis
- ❖ Uterine fibroids

Speak to your doctor before taking Anise if you are currently taking the following prescription or over the counter medications:

- ❖ Some birth control pills

❖ Estrogen pills

Blessed Thistle
(Cnicus benedictus)

❖ Blessed Thistle is sometimes known as *Our Lady's Milk Thistle.*
❖ While not typically considered edible, the leaves, flowers, and stems of Blessed Thistle are often used as a galactagogue to promote lactation and as a compound within some medicinal bitters.
❖ The use of Blessed Thistle dates back to the Middle Ages when it was used to treat the bubonic plague.
❖ Blessed Thistle in tincture form is even mentioned as a cure for the common cold in William Shakespeare's play, *Much Ado about Nothing.*

Blessed Thistle **should not** be taken during pregnancy.

As a non-lactogenic medicinal, Blessed Thistle is often used to treat or prevent the following conditions and illnesses:

❖ Diarrhea
❖ Wounds
❖ Cough
❖ Infections

Precautions to consider before taking Blessed Thistle:

❖ If the recommended dosage is exceeded, Blessed Thistle can cause stomach irritation and vomiting.

Blessed Thistle may cause an allergic reaction in people who suffer from allergies to:

- ❖ Ragweed
- ❖ Chrysanthemums
- ❖ Marigolds
- ❖ Daisies.

Use precaution when taking Blessed Thistle if you are currently being treated for the following disorders:

- ❖ Intestinal infections
- ❖ Chron's Disease

Blessed Thistle may cause the following side effects:

- ❖ Vomiting if taken in excess

Speak to your doctor before taking Blessed Thistle if you are currently taking any of the following prescription or over the counter medications:

- ❖ Tums and Rol-Aids
- ❖ Cimetidine
- ❖ Ranitidine
- ❖ Nizatidine
- ❖ famotidine (Pepcid)
- ❖ Proton pump inhibitors

Borage
(Borago officinalis)

- ❖ Borage is also known as *starflower*.

- ❖ While once grown for culinary and medicinal properties, borage is now commonly cultivated for the oil extracted from its seeds.
- ❖ Borage is often used in gardens as a companion plant because it is known to nurse and protect legumes, spinach, strawberries, and tomatoes.
- ❖ Borage seeds contain about 26 to 38% of natural oil, the richest known source of gamma-linolenic acid (GLA).

Borage may be used to regulate the metabolism and hormonal system, help with PMS, and calm the hot flashes associated with menopause.

Borage **should not** be used during pregnancy.

There are no known allergic reactions or side effects associated with Borage.

As a non-lactogenic medicinal, Borage is often used to treat or prevent the following conditions and illnesses:

- ❖ Hyperactive gastrointestinal disorders
- ❖ Respiratory disorders
- ❖ Cardiovascular disorders
- ❖ Colic
- ❖ Cramps
- ❖ Diarrhea
- ❖ Asthma
- ❖ Bronchitis
- ❖ Kidney and bladder conditions

Borage is sometimes used as:

❖ A diuretic and blood purifier

Precautions to consider before taking Borage:

❖ Borage is not meant to be used on a long-term basis.
❖ Because it contains an alkaloid that can be hard on the liver, it is not one of the herbs that is recommended for nursing mothers or babies.
❖ Pyrrolizidine Alkaloids (PAs) are often unsafe chemicals when taken orally, as they can cause damage to the liver, or even cause cancer, when ingested in high amounts. Borage leaves, flower, and seed can contain PAs, so when using this herb, be sure to do so only if the product has been certified and labeled PA-free.

Use precaution when taking Borage if you are currently being treated for the following disorders:

❖ Bleeding disorders

If you are planning to undergo surgery, stop taking Borage at least two weeks before your medical procedure.

Speak to your doctor before taking Borage if you are currently taking any of the following prescription or over the counter medications:

❖ Carbamazepine
❖ Phenobarbital
❖ Phenytoin
❖ Rifampin

- ❖ Rifabutin
- ❖ Aspirin
- ❖ Clopidogrel
- ❖ Diclofenac
- ❖ Cataflam
- ❖ Ibuprofen (Advil, Motrin, others)
- ❖ Naproxen
- ❖ Dalteparin
- ❖ Enoxaparin
- ❖ Heparin
- ❖ warfarin (Coumadin)
- ❖ NSAIDs

Taking Borage alongside NSAIDs can be toxic.

Caraway
(Carum carvi)

- ❖ Caraway is a member of the carrot family.
- ❖ Caraway seeds are typically used whole, and have a strong black licorice flavor.
- ❖ Finland supplies nearly 30 percent of the world's caraway production.
- ❖ Caraway has been used for culinary and medicinal purposes, as well as a galactagogue to increase and enrich breast milk.

Large doses of Caraway should be avoided during pregnancy.

There are no known allergic reactions associated with Caraway.

As a non-lactogenic medicinal, Caraway is often

used to treat or prevent the following conditions and illnesses:

* Digestive problems
* Heartburn
* Bloating
* Gas
* Loss of appetite
* Mild spasms of the stomach and intestines
* Urination flow
* Blood flow
* Constipation
* Menstrual discomfort

Precautions to consider before taking Caraway:

* Do not take in large doses if you are prone to breast infections.
* Caraway may cause excessive drowsiness.

Use precaution when taking Caraway if you are currently being treated for the following disorders:

* Diabetes
* Hemochromatosis

Caraway may cause the following side effects:

* Belching
* Heartburn, and nausea when used with peppermint oil
* Skin rashes and itching in sensitive people when applied to the skin.

Speak to your doctor before taking Caraway if you are currently taking any of the following prescription or over the counter medications:

- ❖ Glimepiride
- ❖ Glyburide
- ❖ Insulin,
- ❖ Pioglitazone
- ❖ Rosiglitazone
- ❖ Chlorpropamide
- ❖ Glipizide
- ❖ Tolbutamide

Chasteberry
(Vitex agnus-castus)

- ❖ Chasteberry is also called *vitex*.
- ❖ Chasteberry flowers are known to attract butterflies.
- ❖ In ancient times, vitex was believed to be an aphrodisiac.
- ❖ Chasteberry is typically taken as a tincture, decoction, or elixir, and has been used as a galactagogue and as a means of relieving PMS, breast pain, uterine fibroids, and symptoms associated with menopause.

Do not take Chasteberry if you are pregnant.

There are no known allergies associated with Chasteberry.

As a non-lactogenic medicinal, Chasteberry is often used to treat or prevent the following conditions and illnesses:

- ❖ Acne
- ❖ Nervousness
- ❖ Dementia
- ❖ Joint conditions
- ❖ Colds
- ❖ Upset stomach
- ❖ Spleen disorders
- ❖ Headaches
- ❖ Migraine
- ❖ eye pain
- ❖ Body inflammation
- ❖ Swelling.

Precautions to consider before taking Chasteberry:

- ❖ Chasteberry can interfere with the effectiveness of in vitro fertilization.

Use precaution when taking Chasteberry if you are currently being treated for the following disorders:

- ❖ Parkinson's disease
- ❖ Schizophrenia or other mental disorders
- ❖ Endometriosis
- ❖ Uterine fibroids
- ❖ Cancer of the breast, uterus, or ovaries

Chasteberry may cause the following side effects:

- ❖ Upset stomach
- ❖ Nausea
- ❖ Itching
- ❖ Rash

- ❖ Headaches
- ❖ Acne
- ❖ Trouble sleeping
- ❖ Weight gain
- ❖ Change in menstrual flow.

Speak to your doctor before taking Chasteberry if you are currently taking any of the following prescription or over the counter medications:

- ❖ Some birth control pills
- ❖ Some estrogens
- ❖ Chlorpromazine
- ❖ Clozapine
- ❖ Fluphenazine
- ❖ Haloperidol
- ❖ Olanzapine
- ❖ Perphenazine
- ❖ Prochlorperazine
- ❖ Quetiapine
- ❖ Risperidone
- ❖ Thioridazine
- ❖ Thiothixene
- ❖ Bromocriptine
- ❖ Levodopa
- ❖ Pramipexole
- ❖ Ropinirole
- ❖ Raglan

Coriander
(Coriandrum sativum)

- ❖   Coriander is also known as c*ilantro* or *Chinese parsley,* and has a distinct lemon flavor
- ❖ Coriander leaves are extremely rich in vitamins A, C, and K, and contain a moderate content of dietary minerals.
- ❖ Coriander seeds provide significant amounts of dietary fiber, calcium, selenium, iron, magnesium and manganese.

Very little is known regarding the safe use of coriander during pregnancy, so be sure to consult a qualified health care professional before taking this herb if you are pregnant.

There are currently no known medications that negatively interact with Coriander.

As a non-lactogenic medicinal, Coriander is often used to treat or prevent the following conditions amd illnesses:

- ❖ Digestion problems
- ❖ Upset stomach
- ❖ Loss of appetite
- ❖ Nausea
- ❖ Diarrhea
- ❖ Bowel spasms
- ❖ Intestinal gas
- ❖ Measles
- ❖ Hemorrhoids
- ❖ Toothaches
- ❖ Joint pain
- ❖ Infections caused by bacteria and fungus.

Precautions to consider before taking Coriander:

❖ When coming into direct contact with coriander, some people experience skin irritation or inflammation.

Coriander may cause an allergic reaction in people who suffer from allergies to:

❖ Anise
❖ Caraway
❖ Fennel
❖ Dill

Use precaution when taking Coriander if you are currently being treated for the following disorders:

❖ Diabetes
❖ Low blood pressure

Coriander may cause the following side effects:

❖ Increased sensitivity to sunlight
❖ Sunburn
❖ Blistering
❖ Skin rash
❖ Skin cancer

Cumin
(Cuminum cyminum)

❖ Cumin is a member of the parsley family.

- Because of their seed similarities, cumin and coriander are commonly mistaken for one another.
- Cumin seeds are high in iron, and have been used since ancient times for their flavor and medicinal properties.

There are no known allergic reactions or side effects associated with Cumin.

Women who are pregnant should avoid taking large amounts of Cumin.

As a non-lactogenic medicinal, Cumin is often used to treat or prevent the following conditions and illnesses:

- Digestive problems
- Diarrhea
- Colic
- Bowel spasms
- Gas
- Increased urine flow

Cumin may also be used as:

- A diuretic
- A method of prompting the onset of menstruation
- An aphrodisiac

Precautions to consider before taking Cumin:

- Cumin may cause increased drowsiness.
- Large amounts of cumin should be avoided by women who are prone to breast infections.

❖ Avoid taking Cumin at least two weeks before a scheduled surgical procedure.

Use precaution when taking Cumin if you are currently being treated for the following disorders:

Bleeding disorders
Diabetes

Speak to your doctor before taking Cumin if you are currently taking any of the following prescription or over the counter medications:

Glimepiride
Glyburide
Insulin
Pioglitazone
Rosiglitazone
Chlorpropamide
Glipizide
 Tolbutamide

<h3 style="text-align:center">Dandelion Leaf
(Taraxacum officinale)</h3>

❖ In France, the common dandelion is referred to as *dent de lion* because of its jagged "lion tooth" like leaves.
❖ Dandelions are rich in nutrients, containing calcium, iron, magnesium, manganese, phosphorus, potassium, selenium, zinc, vitamins B1, B2, B3 and high amounts of vitamin C and beta-carotene.
❖ The dandelion is said to support the liver, increase

bile production, reduce cholesterol and uric acid levels, and improve the functioning of the kidneys, spleen, pancreas and stomach. It is used for fluid retention, anemia, constipation, abscesses, boils, cirrhosis of the liver, and rheumatism. It is also used in the treatment of hepatitis and jaundice.

❖ In China, varieties of the dandelion have been used since ancient times to treat breast problems such as cancer and mastitis, and for increasing milk production.

❖ Throughout history dandelion was prized for its various medicinal properties, as it contains a wide range of pharmacologically active compounds.

❖ With very low or even no toxicity at all, dandelion can be eaten or taken as a tea on a daily basis.

Because little is known about the safe use of dandelion during pregnancy, it is recommended that pregnant women discuss this herb with their doctor before taking it.

As a non-lactogenic medicinal, Dandelion is often used to treat or prevent the following conditions and illnesses:

❖ Digestive disorders
❖ Infections
❖ Bile and liver disorders

Precautions to consider before taking Dandelion:

❖ Because dandelion acts as a natural diuretic, it should not be taken in conjunction with prescription water pills.

- ❖ Many herbalists recommend that dandelion be taken at the recommended dosage for no longer than three to four weeks at a time.

Dandelion may cause an allergic reaction in people who suffer from allergies to:

- ❖ Ragweed
- ❖ Daisies
- ❖ Chrysanthemums
- ❖ Marigolds

Use precaution when taking Dandelion if you are currently being treated for the following disorders:

- ❖ Obstructed bile ducts
- ❖ Gallbladder disease
- ❖ Gall stones

Speak to your doctor before taking Dandelion if you are currently taking any of the following prescription or over the counter medications:

- ❖ Ciprofloxacin
- ❖ Enoxacin
- ❖ Norfloxacin
- ❖ Sparfloxacin
- ❖ Trovafloxacin
- ❖ Grepafloxacin
- ❖ Lithium.
- ❖ Amitriptyline
- ❖ Haloperidol

- Ondansetron
- Propranolol
- Theophylline
- Verapamil
- Acetaminophen
- Atorvastatin
- Diazepam
- Digoxin
- Entacapone
- Estrogen
- Irinotecan
- Lamotrigine
- Lorazepam
- Lovastatin
- Meprobamate
- Morphine
- Oxazepam
- Water pills

Dill
(Anethum graveolens)

- Dill is very similar to fennel in appearance, and much like caraway in flavor.
- Dill oil is extracted from the leaves, stems and seeds of the plant.
- The ancient Greek doctor, Dioscorides, recommended a decoction of dill to "bring down the milk", probably in reference to the let-down reflex, and a remedy from India uses dill to speed the onset of milk production.

Large amounts of dill should not be taken during pregnancy.

Because Dill is a natural diuretic, it may negatively interact with water pills.

As a non-lactogenic medicinal, Dill is often used to treat or prevent the following conditions and illnesses:

* **Digestive problems**
* **Loss of appetite**
* Intestinal gas
* Liver problems
* Gallbladder problems
* Urinary tract disorder
* Kidney disease
* Painful or difficult urination
* Colds
* Fever
* Cough
* Bronchitis
* Hemorrhoids
* Infection
* Spasms
* Nerve pain
* Genital ulcers
* Menstrual cramps
* Sleep disorders

Precautions you should consider before using Dill:

Women who are prone to breast infections should not

take large amounts of Dill.

Dill may cause an allergic reaction in people who suffer from allergies to:

❖ Celery
❖ Coriander
❖ Caraway
❖ Fennel

Use precaution when taking Dill if you are currently being treated for the following disorders:

❖ Diabetes

Dill nay cause the following side effects:

❖ Skin rash
❖ Sensitivity to sunlight
❖ Sunburn
❖ Blistering

Echinacea
(Echinacea Angustifolia)

❖ Echinacea, commonly called *purple coneflowers*, is one of nine species of plants in the daisy family.
❖ Echinacea can help to prevent nursing inflammations of the breasts, such as engorgement and mastitis, that might otherwise require antibiotics, and is thought to be most effective against breast infection if taken at the first sign of tenderness or redness.

In most cases, Echinacea is considered safe for pregnant women, even during the first trimester of their pregnancy, if taken in small doses; however, it is recommended that expectant mothers consult a qualified medical professional before using any herb or supplement.

As a non-lactogenic medicinal, Echinacea is often used to treat or prevent the following conditions and illnesses:

* The common cold
* Flu
* Upper respiratory infections
* Urinary tract infections
* Vaginal yeast infections
* Herpes
* HIV/AIDS
* Syphilis
* Human Papilloma Virus (HPV).
* Bloodstream infections
* Tonsillitis
* Streptococcus infections
* Typhoid
* Malaria.
* Ear infection
* Swine flu
* Warts
* Anxiety
* Chronic Fatigue Syndrome (CFS)
* Rheumatoid Arthritis
* Migraines
* Acid indigestion

- ❖ Pain
- ❖ Dizziness
- ❖ Attention Deficit-Hyperactivity Disorder (ADHD)

Echinacea is believed to improve the following:

- ❖ Exercise performance

When applied to the skin, Echinacea is used to treat:

- ❖ Boils
- ❖ Gum disease
- ❖ Abscesses
- ❖ Skin wounds
- ❖ Ulcers
- ❖ Burns
- ❖ Eczema
- ❖ Psoriasis
- ❖ Sun-related skin damage
- ❖ Herpes simplex
- ❖ Yeast infections
- ❖ Bee stings.

Precautions to consider before taking Echinacea:

- ❖ Because of concerns that it could exhaust the immune system through over-stimulation, echinacea should not be taken for more than four weeks.
- ❖ It should not be used to treat serious autoimmune diseases.
- ❖ If you suffer from diabetes, it should only be taken under medical supervision.
- ❖ Combining caffeine with echinacea may cause jitters,

headache, and accelerated heartbeat.

Echinacea may cause an allergic reaction in people who suffer from allergies to:

- Ragweed
- Chrysanthemums
- Marigolds
- Daisies

Use precaution when taking Echinacea if you are currently being treated for the following disorders:

- Multiple Sclerosis (MS)
- Lupus
- Rheumatoid Arthritis (RA)
- Pemphigus Vulgaris

Echinacea may cause the following side effects:

- Fever
- Nausea
- Vomiting
- An unpleasant taste in the mouth
- Stomach pain
- Diarrhea
- Sore throat
- Dry mouth
- Headache
- Numbness of the tongue
- Dizziness
- Insomnia
- Disorientation

❖   Joint and muscle aches

Applying echinacea to the skin may cause redness, itchiness, or a rash.

Speak to your doctor before taking Echinacea if you are currently taking any of the following prescription or over the counter medications:

❖   Lovastatin
❖   Cyclosporine
❖   Diltiazem
❖   Estrogens,
❖   Indinavir
❖   Triazolam
❖   Cyclobenzaprine
❖   Fluvoxamine
❖   Haloperidol
❖   Imipramine
❖   Mexiletine
❖   Olanzapine
❖   Pentazocine
❖   Propranolol
❖   Tacrine
❖   Theophylline
❖   Zileuton
❖   Zolmitriptan

Or immunosuppressants such as:

❖   Azathioprine
❖   Basiliximab
❖   Cyclosporine
❖   Daclizumab

- ❖ Muromonab-CD3
- ❖ Orthoclone
- ❖ Mycophenolate
- ❖ Tacrolimus
- ❖ Sirolimus
- ❖ Prednisone
- ❖ Corticosteroids

* Midazolam **may** negatively interact with Echinacea.

Fennel
(Foeniculum vulgare)

- ❖ The name *Fennel* derives from the Middle English word *fenyl*.
- ❖ Fennel is highly regarded as a galactagogue, and when taken at a high dosage for a few days, its seeds can dramatically increase milk supply.
- ❖ Fennel seed is a common ingredient in lactation herbal mixtures. It can be taken alone as a "single," or used alongside other lactogenics.

Fennel is considered an estrogenic herb, and precautions should be taken when using it in with other estrogens.

Pregnant women should avoid taking large amounts of fennel.

As a non-lactogenic medicinal, Fennel is often used to treat or prevent the following conditions or illnesses:

- ❖ Heartburn
- ❖ Intestinal gas

- ❖ Bloating
- ❖ Loss of appetite
- ❖ Colic in infants
- ❖ Upper respiratory tract infections
- ❖ Coughs
- ❖ Bronchitis
- ❖ Cholera backache
- ❖ Vision problems

Precautions to consider before taking Fennel:

- ❖ In Traditional Chinese Medicine, fennel seed is said to have a drying quality that will reduce milk production if taken at a high dosage over a long period of time.

Fennel may cause an allergic reaction in people who suffer from allergies to:

- ❖ Celery
- ❖ Carrots

Use precaution when taking Fennel if you are currently being treated for the following disorders:

- ❖ Bleeding disorders
- ❖ Breast cancer
- ❖ Uterine cancer
- ❖ Ovarian cancer
- ❖ Endometriosis
- ❖ Uterine fibroids

Speak to your doctor before taking Fennel if you are currently taking any of the following prescription or

over the counter medications:

* Some birth control pills
* Some estrogens

Do not take fennel if you are taking tamoxifen.
Ciprofloxacin **may** negatively interact with fennel.

Fenugreek
(Trigonella foenum-graecum)

* While Fenugreek seeds contain hormone precursors that increase breast milk supply, scientists still aren't clear why this happens. Some theorize that it may occur because breasts are modified sweat glands and Fenugreek is known to stimulate sweat production.
* It has been shown that Fenugreek can increase a nursing woman's breast milk supply within 24-72 hours, and that once an adequate lactation level has been achieved, most women can discontinue taking the herb and maintain their supply with proper breast stimulation and milk removal.
* Fenugreek has long been known to be effective as a natural breast enlarger, as the herb's diosgenin are used to make synthetic estrogen that has been shown to cause growth in breast cells.
* The herb may also help to increase sexual desire and improve the breasts' overall beauty and health.
* Fenugreek also contains choline, which may aid in the thinking process, and antioxidants that slow aging and help to prevent disease.
* Fenugreek contains a very potent aromatic compound called solotone, which gives this herb its distinct maple syrup scent.

Though most women respond quickly to Fenugreek seed tea, capsules, or tinctures, not every woman does. Some see more success when taking Fenugreek in combination with other lactogenic herbs.

Fenugreek should not be taken during pregnancy.

As a non-lactogenic medicinal, Echinacea is often used to treat or prevent the following conditions and illnesses:

- Loss of appetite
- Upset stomach
- Constipation
- Gastritis
- Diabetes
- Painful menstruation
- Polycystic Ovary Syndrome
- Obesity
- Atherosclerosis
- High cholesterol
- High triglycerides
- Kidney ailments
- Mouth ulcers
- Boils
- Bronchitis
- Cellulitis
- Tuberculosis
- Chronic coughs
- Chapped lips
- Baldness
- Cancer
- Parkinson's disease

Fenugreek is also thought to improve the following:

Exercise performance.

Precautions to consider before taking Fenugreek:

❖ Fenugreek must be taken consistently to avoid a decrease in breast milk supply.

Fenugreek may cause an allergic reaction in people who suffer from allergies to:

❖ Soybeans
❖ Peanuts
❖ Legumes
❖ Green peas

Use precaution when taking Echinacea if you are currently being treated for the following disorders:

❖ Diabetes

Fenugreek can cause hypoglycemia.
Consult your doctor before taking Fenugreek if you are taking any blood-thinning medications.

Fenugreek may cause the following side effects:

❖ A maple syrup aroma on the skin, in perspiration, breast milk, and other bodily fluids.
❖ Diarrhea
❖ Stomach upset
❖ Bloating

❖ Gas

Unless a person experiences hypersensitivity to this herb, these side effects typically disappear within a few days after the dosage has begun.

Speak to your doctor before taking Fenugreek if you are currently taking any of the following prescription or over the counter medications:

❖ Gimepiride
❖ Glyburide
❖ Insulin
❖ Pioglitazone
❖ Rosiglitazone
❖ Chlorpropamide
❖ Glipizide
❖ Tolbutamide
❖ Aspirin
❖ Clopidogrel
❖ Diclofenac
❖ Ibuprofen
❖ Naproxen
❖ Dalteparin
❖ Enoxaparin
❖ Heparin.
❖ Warfarin (Coumadin)

Garlic
(Allium sativumarlic)

❖ Garlic is closely related to the onion, shallot, leek, and chive.

❖   Along with properties that may ease everything from the common cold to certain types of cancer, garlic is also used as a galactogogue.

As a non-lactogenic medicinal, Garlic is often used to treat or prevent the following conditions and illnesses:

❖   High blood pressure
❖   Low blood pressure
❖   High cholesterol
❖   Inherited high cholesterol
❖   Coronary heart disease
❖   Heart attack
❖   Reduced blood flow due to narrowed arteries Atherosclerosis
❖   Colon cancer
❖   Rectal cancer
❖   Stomach cancer
❖   Breast cancer
❖   Prostate cancer
❖   Multiple myeloma
❖   Lung cancer
❖   Enlarged prostate
❖   Cystic fibrosis
❖   Diabetes
❖   Osteoarthritis
❖   Hay fever
❖   Pre-eclampsia
❖   Yeast infection
❖   Flu
❖   Bacterial and fungal infections
❖   Earaches

* Chronic fatigue syndrome
* Menstrual disorders
* Abnormal cholesterol levels caused by HIV drugs
* Hepatitis
* Shortness of breath related to liver disease
* Stomach ulcers
* Fibrocystic breast disease
* Fever
* Cough
* Headaches
* Stomach aches
* Sinus congestion
* Gout
* Joint pain
* Hemorrhoids
* Asthma
* Bronchitis
* Low blood sugar
* Tooth sensitivity
* Gastritis
* Stress
* Fatigue

Garlic may also be used to improve:

Exercise performance

Precautions to consider before taking Garlic:

* When taken in high doses, garlic can cause bad breath and body odor, and can transfer into breast milk, giving it a strong and unpleasant aroma that can pass to the nursing partner.

Garlic may cause an allergic reaction in people who suffer from allergies to:

- ❖ Hyacinth
- ❖ Tulip
- ❖ Onion
- ❖ Leek
- ❖ Chives

Use precaution when taking Echinacea if you are currently being treated for the following disorders:

Bleeding disorders
Stomach and digestive problems
Low blood pressure

Garlic may cause the following side effects:

- ❖ A burning sensation in the mouth or stomach
- ❖ Heartburn
- ❖ Gas
- ❖ Diarrhea
- ❖ Nausea
- ❖ Vomiting

When applied directly to the skin, raw garlic can cause rash or irritation.

Speak to your doctor before taking Echinacea if you are currently taking any of the following prescription or over the counter medications:

- ❖ Isoniazid

- Cyclosporine
- Delavirdine
- Efavirenz
- Some estrogen-containing birth control pills
- Acetaminophen
- Chlorzoxazone
- Ethanol
- Theophylline
- Drugs used for anesthesia during surgery
- Warfarin (Coumadin)

Goat's Rue
(Galega officinalis)

- Also known as *Holy Hay* and *French lilac*, the name Goat's Rue derives from the word *gala* (meaning *milk*) and *ago* (meaning (*to bring on.*)
- Goat's Rue is typically used in conjunction with its sister herb Fenugreek to maximize its lactogenic efficiency.

Although goat's rue is considered somewhat controversial, it remains a popular lactogenic herb for many women , and because very few problems associated with the consumption of this galactagogue have been reported, experienced herbalists are generally quite comfortable with recommending it as a supplement.

Goat's rue seems to be particularly beneficial to women who experience insufficient glandular tissue of the breast. While mild amounts of Goat's Rue are thought to be relatively safe for most pregnant women, it is better to consult a qualified health care professional before taking this herb if you are currently expecting a child.

As a non-lactogenic medicinal, Goat's Rue is often used to treat or prevent the following illnesses:

- ❖ Stimulation of the adrenal glands and pancreas
- ❖ Diabetes
- ❖ Digestive problems

Goat's Rue is also used as a diuretic and blood purifier.

Precautions to consider before taking Goat's Rue:

- ❖ **Do not** confuse it with rue.
- ❖ While fresh Goat's Rue is considered toxic, the dried variety is considered safe for use in tinctures or teas.
- ❖ People currently being treated for diabetes should only use Goat's Rue under a doctor's supervision.

Goat's Rue may cause an allergic reaction in people who suffer from allergies to:

- ❖ Soybeans
- ❖ Peanuts
- ❖ Legumes
- ❖ Green peas

Use precaution when taking Echinacea if you are currently being treated for the following disorders:

- ❖ Blood disorders

Speak to your doctor before taking Echinacea if you are currently taking any of the following prescription

or over the counter medications:

- ❖ Glimepiride
- ❖ Glyburide
- ❖ Insulin
- ❖ Pioglitazone
- ❖ Chlorpropamide
- ❖ Glipizide
- ❖ Tolbutamide

Hops
(Humulus lupulus)

- ❖ Hops cultivation first began in the United States in the 1600s.
- ❖ For generations, hops have been used in herbal medicines as a treatment for anxiety, restlessness, and insomnia.
- ❖ Hops give beer its amber color and bitter taste.
- ❖ Hops is an estrogenic relaxant, and in folk medicine, pillows were stuffed with hops flowers to promote sleep.
- ❖ It is believed that hops may help to trigger the nursing woman's let-down reflex.

When taken as a bitter tea, hops is often used to begin the flow of breast milk.

Hops can cause a variety of allergic reactions, including skin rash and severe irritation, in hypersensitive people. Hops is **highly** hormonal and **should be avoided** during pregnancy.

As a non-lactogenic medicinal, Hops is often used to

treat or prevent the following conditions and illnesses:

- ❖ ADHD
- ❖ Nervousness
- ❖ Excitability
- ❖ Irritability
- ❖ Indigestion
- ❖ Cancers of the prostate, breast, and ovaries
- ❖ High cholesterol
- ❖ Tuberculosis
- ❖ Bladder infection
- ❖ Intestinal cramps
- ❖ Colitis
- ❖ Nerve pain

Hops may also be used to:

- ❖ Relieve tension
- ❖ Improve appetite
- ❖ Increase urine flow

Precautions to consider before taking Hops:

- ❖ Hops **should not** be used if you suffer from depression.
- ❖ Hops can act as a sedative, causing drowsiness or lethargy, so exercise precaution when using this as a supplement.
- ❖ Alcoholic beverages can negatively interact with hops.

Use precaution when taking Echinacea if you are

currently being treated for the following disorders:

* Breast cancer
* Endometriosis

Hops may cause the following side effects:

* Depression
* Lethargy

Speak to your doctor before taking Hops if you are currently taking any of the following prescription or over the counter medications:

* Clonazepam
* Lorazepam
* Phenobarbital
* Zolpidem

Marshmallow Root and Leaf
(Althaea officinalis)

* The traditional medicinal uses of the Marshmallow plant are reflected in the name of the genus, which comes from the Greek , meaning "to heal", and was used in ancient Egypt as a remedy for sore throats.
* Marshmallow root is also a Native American galactagogue, often used in combination with Fenugreek, Red Clover, Alfalfa, or Blessed Thistle.
* Marshmallow contains mucilage, a substance that can soothe and calm inflammation in the intestines, stomach, upper respiratory tract, throat, and mouth.

There are currently no known allergic reactions or side

effects associated with Marshmallow Root.

Pregnant women should speak to a qualified health care professional before taking this herb.

As a non-lactogenic medicinal, Marshmallow Root and Leaf are often used to treat or prevent the following conditions and illnesses:

* Inflammation of the respiratory tract
* Dry cough
* Inflammation of the stomach lining
* Diarrhea
* Stomach ulcers
* Constipation
* Urinary tract infection
* Kidney stones

Marshmallow Root is sometimes used as an ingredient in skin ointments to relieve:

* Chapped skin
* Swelling and pain of the feet and hands due to exposure to the cold
* Skin infections
* Burns
* Wounds

Precautions to consider before taking Marshmallow Root:

* **Do not** confuse this herb with the mallow (Malva sylvestris) flower and leaf.
* Marshmallow root, which acts as a diuretic, may also

affect how quickly the body absorbs other medications, so be cautious when using it with prescription medications.

❖ If you take Lithium, consult your doctor before taking marshmallow root and leaf.

Use precaution when taking Marshmallow Root and Leaf if you are currently being treated for the following disorders:

❖ Diabetes

Marshmallow Root may cause a significant drop in blood sugar levels, particularly before or following surgical procedures.

Speak to your doctor before taking Echinacea if you are currently taking any of the following prescription or over the counter medications:

❖ Glimepiride
❖ Glyburide
❖ Insulin
❖ Pioglitazone
❖ Chlorpropamide
❖ Glipizide
❖ Tolbutamide

Nettle Leaf
(Urtica dioica)

❖ Nettle can be easily found throughout Canada and in

every state of the U.S. except Hawaii.
❖ The plant parts, both underground roots and above ground leaves, are edible, and have a long history of valued medicinal properties.
❖ Nettle is a good source of calcium and iron, magnesium, manganese, phosphorus, potassium, selenium, sulfur, zinc, copper, chlorophyll, fatty acids, and folate as well as vitamins K, B1, B2, B3, B5, C, and E.
❖ Nettle is useful in the treatment of iron deficiency.

Allergic reactions to nettle are very rare.

Pregnant women should speak to a qualified medical professional before using nettle leaf.

As a non-lactogenic medicinal, Nettle Leaf is often used to treat or prevent the following illnesses:

Joint ailments,
Anemia
Poor circulation
Diabetes
Stomach acidity
Lung congestion
Rash
Eczema
Cancer
Wounds
Enlarged spleen

Stinging Nettle is also used as a diuretic and blood purifier, an astringent, to control uterine bleeding, and prevent the signs of aging.

Precautions to consider before taking Nettle Leaf:

❖ Do not confuse stinging nettle with white dead nettle (Lamium album).
❖ Because this herb acts as a diuretic, it may alter how effectively the body absorbs some medications.

Use precaution when taking Echinacea if you are currently being treated for the following disorders:

❖ Diabetes
❖ Low blood pressure

Nettle Leaf may cause the following side effects:

Stomach or digestive upsets
Increased sweating
Drowsiness

Speak to your doctor before taking Nettle Leaf if you are currently taking any of the following prescription or over the counter medications:

❖ Glimepiride
❖ Insulin
❖ Pioglitazone
❖ Rosiglitazone
❖ Chlorpropamide
❖ Glipizide
❖ Tolbutamide
❖ Captopril
❖ Enalapril
❖ Losartan

- Valsartan
- Diltiazem
- Amlodipine
- Hydrochlorothiazide
- Furosemide
- Clonazepam
- Lorazepam
- Phenobarbital
- Zolpidem (Ambien).
- Lithium
- Warfarin (Coumadin)

Red Clover
(Trifolium pratense)

- Red Clover is a member of the bean family, and is highly nutritious.
- In traditional medicine, Red Clover has been used to move obstructions in the body and ease spasms.
- It is also used as a sedative, an anti-inflammatory, and as a means of treating some skin conditions.
- As a galactagogue, Red Clover flowers are often used along with Fenugreek, Alfalfa, and Blessed Thistle to promote lactation.
- Fresh Red Clover flowers are edible, and often used in salads.

Allergic reactions are rare when red clover is taken in recommended dosages.

Because red clover is estrogenic, pregnant women should consult a qualified health care professional before using it.

As a non-lactogenic medicinal, Red Clover is often

used to treat or prevent the following conditions and illnesses:

- ❖ Cancer
- ❖ Indigestion
- ❖ High cholesterol
- ❖ Cough
- ❖ Asthma
- ❖ Bronchitis
- ❖ Wounds
- ❖ Burns
- ❖ Eczema
- ❖ Psoriasis
- ❖ Breast pain
- ❖ PMS
- ❖ Hot flashes

Precautions to consider before taking Echinacea:

Red clover may cause excessive drowsiness or lethargy.

Use precaution when taking Echinacea if you are currently being treated for the following disorders:

- ❖ Bleeding disorders
- ❖ Breast cancer
- ❖ Uterine cancer
- ❖ Ovarian cancer
- ❖ Endometriosis
- ❖ Blood clots
- ❖ Protein S deficiency

Red clover may also cause prolonged bleeding during and

after surgery, so it is recommended that its use be stopped at least two weeks prior to any scheduled surgical procedures.

Red Clover may cause the following side effects:

❖ Rash
❖ Muscle aches
❖ Headaches
❖ Nausea
❖ Vaginal bleeding (spotting)

Speak to your doctor before taking Red Clover if you are currently taking any of the following prescription or over the counter medications:

❖ Some estrogen-containing birth control
❖ Estrogen pills
❖ Amitriptyline
❖ Haloperidol
❖ Ondansetron
❖ Propranolol
❖ Theophylline
❖ Verapamil
❖ Omeprazole
❖ Lansoprazole
❖ Pantoprazole
❖ Diazepam
❖ Carisoprodol
❖ Nelfinavir
❖ Diclofenac
❖ Ibuprofen
❖ Meloxicam

- Piroxicam
- Celecoxib
- Amitriptyline
- Warfarin
- Glipizide
- Losartan
- Lovastatin
- Ketoconazole
- Itraconazole
- Fexofena
- Triazolam
- Aspirin
- Clopidogrel
- Diclofenac
- Cataflam
- Ibuprofen
- Naproxen
- Dalteparin
- Enoxaparin
- Heparin
- Warfarin (Coumadin)
- Tamoxifen

Red Raspberry Leaf
(Rubus Idaeus)

- Native Americans gave raspberry leaves to women during childbirth to strengthen and speed delivery.
- Red raspberry leaf tea provides an excellent source of minerals and vitamins and, as a lactogenic herb, may help build breast tissue, and encourage and enrich breast milk supply.

Allergic reactions to red raspberry are very rare, and there are no known side effects or medication interactions associated with this herb.

Because red raspberry tea may stimulate the uterus, during pregnancy, if you are using Red Raspberry Leaf as a tea, it is important to build up dosage slowly. To be certain that Red Raspberry Leaf is safe for you, consult a qualified medical professional prior to using this herb, particularly if you are at risk for miscarriage.

As a non-lactogenic medicinal, Red Raspberry Leaf is often used to treat or prevent the following conditions and illnesses:

- ❖ Digestive problems
- ❖ Heart problems
- ❖ Respiratory system disorders
- ❖ Diabetes
- ❖ vitamin deficiencies
- ❖ Fluid retention
- ❖ Skin rash
- ❖ Sore throat.

Precautions to consider before taking Red Raspberry Leaf:

Raspberry leaf tea is an astringent, which tightens and constricts body tissues, so when taken alone for longer than two weeks, it can act as an anti-lactogenic by decreasing breast milk supply. It is recommended that red raspberry leaf be taken as an ingredient in herbal teas and/or tinctures, in conjunction with other lactogenic herbs.

Use precaution when taking Red Raspberry Leaf if you are currently being treated for the following disorders:

❖ Breast cancer
❖ Uterine cancer
❖ Ovarian cancer
❖ Endometriosis
❖ Uterine fibroids

Vervain
(Verbena - Various Species)

❖ Vervain is also called *Verbena or lemon verbena*, and has a long history as an estrogenic herb and health tonic.
❖ Vervain was a holy herb of women in ancient days, known for its divinity.
❖ It was called "tears of Isis" in ancient Egypt, and later called "Hera's tears" in ancient Greece.
❖ Because of its beauty, Vervain is often used as a popular ornamental garden plant known to attract various species of butterflies and hummingbirds.
❖ Verbena is calming, mood-lifting, and is said to prevent depression from developing. It is particularly useful after a viral infection, such as a cold or flu, to prevent exhaustion from lingering, and to restore strength.
❖ All species of verbena are believed to promote milk production.
❖ Vervain is thought to fortify the nerves, alleviate menstrual cramps and the effects of menopause, and help with irregular menstrual bleeding.

Because it is unclear how verbena may affect the uterus, it **should not** be taken during pregnancy.

While there is no known medication interactions related to the use of Vervain, speak to your doctor before taking it if you are currently taking any prescription or over the counter medications.

As a non-lactogenic medicinal, Vervain is often used to treat or prevent the following conditions and illnesses:

- Asthma
- Angina
- Tension headaches
- Gallbladder pain and disease
- Arthritis
- Gout
- Metabolic disorders
- Anemia
- Fever
- Pain
- Spasms
- Exhaustion
- Nervous conditions
- Digestive disorders
- Liver disease
- Jaundice
- Kidney and lower urinary tract disorders

Vervain is sometimes applied directly to the skin as a method of treating:

- ❖ Poorly healing wounds
- ❖ Abscesses
- ❖ Burns
- ❖ Arthritis and joint pain
- ❖ Dislocations
- ❖ Bone bruises
- ❖ Itching.

Precautions to consider before taking Vervain:

- ❖ Verbena may interfere in the action of medications used to treat blood pressure conditions, or those used as hormone therapy.
- ❖ Although traditionally a galactagogue, Traditional Chinese Medicine sees verbena as having a drying property that may decrease milk supply if over-used.

Vervain may cause the following allergic reactions:

Skin rash

Use precaution when taking Vervain if you are currently being treated for the following disorders:

- ❖ Low or high blood pressure
- ❖ Hormone-sensitive conditions.

Vervain may cause the following side effects:

- ❖ Digestive system upset in sensitive people

Chapter 3
Umbel Seeds

In botany, an *inflorescence* is the flowering part of a plant, or the arrangement of flowers on a stalk, also called a *pedicel*. The Umbelliferae species of plants, which contains members of the parsley family, such as dill, coriander, and cumin, are characterized by their small flat or rounded cluster of flowers that grow and spread from the same point in the main stem and have stalks of the same length, giving them an equal and uniform appearance. These small groups are linked to a still larger stem, forming bigger clusters of flowers, with the youngest flowers positioned in the center. In traditional medicine, umbels are said to have an affinity for breasts, and the shape of the umbel reminds some of milk glands, connected by milk ducts to the areola; these look-alike factors can play a role in the historic belief that a plant has certain effects on the body. However, in the case of umbel seeds, experience through use proves that they do indeed increase breast milk supply and improve the let-down reflex. Umbel flowers produce tiny aromatic seeds that can be used as very effective galactagogues. Because some umbel plants and seeds are toxic, wild foraging and harvesting is not recommended.

Every umbel seed is estrogenic and shares the same medicinal and nutritive properties; they promote relaxation, acting as a natural sedative, even as they support digestion, and act as anti-spasmodics to aid in treating bronchitis and asthma.

While they are very effective when used alone, as a single, umbel seeds are a perfect choice for a potent lactogenic or medicinal infusion or decoction, as they can safely be used together in a variety of combinations.

Anise, caraway, coriander, cumin, dill, and fennel are umbel seeds, and make wonderful options for women in search of lactogenic herbs that can be combined into one effective blend to promote lactation, enrich breast milk, and help with let-down for more successful breastfeeding.

Taking large amounts of umbel seeds during pregnancy is not recommended, and these lactogenics may not be suitable for women who are prone to breast infections or eczema. Because each specific seed carries its own allergic reactions and medication interaction precautions, it is important to read about each one prior to its use, to ensure if a certain umbel seed is right for you.

Umbel seeds can be taken individually, together, or combined with other herbs to make a lactation tea. They can be infused overnight in cold or hot water, and make an ideal decoction.

Don't be afraid to experiment! Umbel seeds are a wonderful way for the budding herbalist to concoct their own effective lactogenic or medicinal blend, and craft a one of a kind brew that works perfectly for them!

Chapter 4
Methods of Taking Lactogenic Herbs

There are many ways to take galactagogues as a means of increasing breast milk production and flow, and some methods are more effective than others, as they allow the lactogenic aid to pass more quickly into the blood stream. No matter your preferred method, remember that no herb's potency is immediate; some take several days--or even weeks--to produce results. Be patient. Take the desired galactagogues according to dosage recommendations, and be sure to combine them with more traditional lactation inducing and promoting techniques to ensure their milk-making magic.

Supplements:

Taking galactagogues as an herbal supplement, typically in capsule form, is a popular choice for many women, as taking oral medications is quite easy and convenient. Capsules are often slow to release the herb's medicinal properties, so taking lactogenic aids in supplement form may inhibit their initial effectiveness. Supplements do often work; it just takes a bit longer for women to see results.

Rather than purchasing pre-packaged supplements, some women prefer to prepare their own galactagogues by filling empty capsules with dried herbs. If doing this, it is important to measure herbs carefully, to ensure that each capsule is filled with the correct dosage.

When purchasing herbs, the most healthy--and often most effective--ones are sold in health food stores and herbal shops.

Teas:

Galactagogues can quickly and easily be prepared as teas by steeping one herb--or a combination of herbs--in boiling water. Most lactation teas can be enjoyed throughout the day as a way to boost breast milk supply. Teas can be very effective, but need to be taken regularly and frequently to maximize their potency. A typical dose is three cups of tea per day.

Unfortunately, many herbs have an unpleasant or even butter taste in liquid form, and while some teas can be sweetened or flavored with lemon to improve their taste, others, such as those made from blessed thistle, are identified as *digestive bitters,* and it is that bitterness that aids in the herb's medicinal properties. Bitters should only be moderately sweetened. When flavoring lactation teas, it is better to use natural sweeteners, like honey or stevia, rather than granulated sugar or artificial sweeteners that often contain aspartame.

It is sometimes easier to make a larger batch of tea to drink throughout the day rather than preparing individual cups. If you choose to do this, you can store the left-over tea in the refrigerator; just be sure to drink it within 36 hours to avoid spoilage.

When preparing herbal lactation teas, be sure to pour boiling water over the herbs instead of combining the water and herbs, and then heating them together in the microwave. This quick microwave method of preparing tea reduces the herb's effectiveness.

Many herbs have a specific steeping time. Five minutes of brewing is a great rule of thumb to start with. The longer an herb is stepped, the stronger the tea will be. Shorter steeping times produce a weaker and less effective lactogenic.

Infusion Method:

An infusion is simply a large amount of tea brewed for a long time. Herbal infusions began in Europe, and are now becoming a popular method of preparing a variety of health tonics. Galactagogues can also be prepared as an infusion.

To make an infusion, one cup of dried herbs is placed inside a quart jar, which is then filled to the top with boiling water. The jar is tightly covered, and the herbs are allowed to steep for several hours or overnight. After it has brewed, the infusion is strained, and the liquid is taken as a tea. Because the drying process provides for the preservation of valuable nutrients and medicinal properties, dried herbs make perfect infusions.

To heat a cup of infusion, you should gently warm it in a pan on top of the stove over low heat. You can then sweeten it to taste before drinking it as a tea. The remaining infusion should be refrigerated and used within 36 hours. If any infusion is left after this period of time, discard it and make a fresh batch. A typical dose of infusion is three cups per day.

Cold Infusion Method:

In some countries, herbalists feel that, during the

traditional preparation of an infusion, some of the herbs' nutritive properties are lost to steam and evaporation, so their infusions are prepared cold.

As with the heated infusion method, one cup of dried herbs is placed inside a quart jar, which is then filled to the top with cold water. The jar is tightly covered, and the herbs are allowed to steep for several hours or overnight. After it has brewed, the infusion is strained, and the liquid is taken as a tea.

The infusion can be taken cold, or you can gently warm it per cup in a pan on the stove top over low heat. As with the heated infusion method, the cold infusion can be naturally sweetened to taste, and any remaining brew should be stored in the refrigerator and discarded after 36 hours.

Decoction:

Decoctions have been prepared since ancient times as a way of extracting the medicinal properties from dried herbs. The word *decoct* simply means to simmer for a very long time, and that is what happens when a health tonic is prepared in this way.

To make a decoction, place a pint of water in a pan, and add one cup of herbs to it. Begin to warm them on the stove top over low heat. Do not cover the pan during the process. Continue to simmer the decoction until approximately 1/4 of the water evaporates, and then remove from heat and allow to cool.

Once cooled, strain the herbs and reserve the remaining liquid. You can drink a cup of the decoction cold, or warm it in the same way you would warm a traditional infusion. It can be sweetened naturally to taste. Store the remaining decoction in the rerigerator for up to 36 hours.

Some roots and flowers, such as dandelions and red clover, extract very well in this preparation method, and retain the highest medicinal and nutritive properties. A blend of umbel seeds also make the perfect decoction.

Tinctures:

A tinctures is a really effective way of ingesting a galactagogue, as this method extracts an herb's medicinal and nutritive properties over a lengthy period of time, preserving its quality and effectiveness. Tinctures are typically prepared by extracting herbs through a vegetable glycerin or alcohol base (which, in most cases, is a better choice, as many herbs respond to and draw better from an alcohol base), and because they are taken under the tongue in a specific number of drops, it is believed that the medicine moves into the bloodstream more quickly, so the benefits and health properties are noticed sooner than through other ingestion methods. Although this is a really quick and convenient way to take a galactagogue, tinctures typically have a very unpleasant taste.

Depending on who prepares the tincture and where they are purchased from, you may be instructed to take the tincture by the dropperful, in milliliters, or by a certain number of drops. The dosage is generally repeated two to three times per day for maximum effectiveness.

Tinctures can be diluted in a spoonful of water, or even prepared as an herbal tea, without compromising their effectiveness. To prepare a cup of tea, add the recommended tincture dosage to one cup of boiling water, and lightly sweeten with a natural sweetener, or add lemon to flavor it. Drink three cups of "tincture tea" per day.

When extracted through alcohol, tinctures have an indefinite shelf life, while tinctures prepared through the glycerin method should be discarded after three months.

Chapter 5
Herb Dosage and Preparation

When using herbs for their lactogenic and medicinal properties, it is very important to follow both dosage recommendations and guidelines for the proper preparations of teas, light beverages, elixirs, tinctures, infusions, and decoctions. Following daily dosage suggestions provides a safe and effective way for you to reap the healing and nutritive properties of any plant, root, leaf, flower, or seed, and because each concoction works differently, depending on how it is blended, brewed, and consumed, understanding proper preparation methods can also ensure the potency of your lactogenics and medicinals.

Alfalfa Tea:

Add one to two teaspoons of dried alfalfa to one cup of boiling water. Drink up to three cups of tea per day, or to kick-start milk supply, drink up to six cups of tea per day for several days. An increase in milk supply may be noticeable within two to four days.

Alfalfa Infusion:

Add one to two handfuls of dried alfalfa to a one quart jar of boiling water. Cover the jar tightly, and allow to steep for 10 hours, or over night, before drinking.

As a supplement in capsule form, take up to 60 grams daily.

Anise Tea:

Gently crush one to two teaspoons of anise seeds, and cover them with one cup of boiling water. Cover the cup and steep for five to 20 minutes. Sweeten to taste. Drink three cups of tea per day, or to kick start milk production, drink up to six cups of anise tea for two to four days.

Anise Infusion:

Place one cup of anise seeds in a quart jar of boiling water. Cover the jar and allow to steep for a minimum of four hours before drinking.

As a lactogenic in tincture form, take 3.5 to 7 grams daily.

Blessed Thistle Tea:

Pour a cup of boiling water over one to two teaspoons of dried blessed thistle. Steep for five to 20 minutes. Drink three cups of tea per day, before meals or snacks. To kick-start lactation, you may drink up to five cups of tea per day.

As a supplement in capsule form, take up 2 grams of Blessed Thistle daily.

Blessed thistle can be taken in conjunction with

Fenugreek.

Because it is considered a "bitter", Blessed Thistle should be taken bitter for maximum effectiveness. Don't over-sweeten Blessed Thistle tea.

Borage Tea:

Pour one cup of boiling water over one to two teaspoons of dried borage. Allow to steep for 10 to 15 minutes. Sweeten to taste. Drink up to two cups of tea per day.

Caraway Tea:

Gently crush one to two teaspoons of caraway seeds, and add one cup of boiling water. Cover the cup and steep for five to 20 minutes. Longer steeping time produces a more potent tea. Sweeten to taste.

Light Caraway Tea:

Follow the directions as above, but steep for only one to three minutes for a milder taste and effect.

Caraway Infusion:

Place a handful of caraway seeds in a quart jar and cover with boiling water. Cover jar tightly and allow to steep for a minimum of four hours before drinking.

Cold Caraway Infusion:

Place a handful of caraway seeds in a quart of cold water

and soak them overnight. The following day, strain the liquid and gently warm it on a stove top before drinking. Cold infusion ensures that none of the herb's volatile, medicinal oil is lost to steam.

The usual recommended dosage of Caraway Teas and Infusions is three cups per day. To increase milk production, take up to six cups a day initially, as necessary, but be sure to observe your reaction to this supplement. If you experience any side effects, reduce the dosage, or discontinue use, and consider using a different galactagogue.

Chasteberry Elixir:

Chasteberry remains a controversial lactogenic herb, and should not be taken for long periods of time. The recommended dosage is 35 to 40 milligrams per day, taken as an elixir in the morning.

To prepare a Chasteberry elixir, mix equal parts chasteberry and water and drink. Take no more than the recommended dosage per day.

Coriander Tea:

Gently crush one to two teaspoons of coriander seeds, and add one cup of boiling water. Cover the cup and steep for five to 20 minutes. Longer steeping produces a more potent tea. Sweeten to taste.

Light Coriander Tea:

Follow the directions as above, but steep for only one to

three minutes for a milder taste and effect.

Coriander Infusion:

Place a handful of coriander seeds in a quart jar and cover with boiling water. Cover the jar tightly and allow to steep for a minimum of four hours before drinking.

Cold Coriander Infusion:

Placed a handful of coriander seeds in a quart of cold water and soak them overnight. The following day, strain the liquid and gently warm it on a stove top before drinking. Cold infusion ensures that none of the herb's volatile, medicinal oil is lost to steam.

The usual recommended dosage of Coriander Teas and Infusions is three cups per day. To increase milk production, take up to six cups a day initially, as necessary, but be sure to observe your reaction to this supplement,. If you experience any side effects, reduce the dosage, or discontinue use, and consider using a different galactagogue.

Cumin Tea:

Gently crush one to two teaspoons of cumin seeds, and add one cup of boiling water. Cover the cup and steep for five to 20 minutes. Longer steeping produces a more potent tea. Sweeten to taste.

Light Cumin Tea:

Follow the directions as above, but steep for only one to three minutes for a milder taste and effect.

Cumin Infusion:

Place a handful of cumin seeds in a quart jar and cover with boiling water. Cover the jar tightly and allow to steep for a minimum of four hours before drinking.

Cold Cumin Infusion:

Placed a handful of cumin seeds in a quart of cold water and soak them overnight. The following day, strain the liquid and gently warm it on a stove top before drinking. Cold infusion ensures that none of the herb's volatile, medicinal oil is lost to steam.

The usual recommended dosage of Cumin Teas and Infusions is three cups per day. To increase milk production, take up to six cups a day initially, as necessary, but be sure to observe your reaction to this supplement,. If you experience any side effects, reduce the dosage, or discontinue use, and consider using a different galactagogue.

Fresh Dandelion Medicinal:

If dandelions grow naturally near you, and are not exposed to pollution or pesticides, try eating a few of the leaves every day for their support of your milk supply. Dandelion leaves can be eaten whole, chopped and sautéed in virgin olive oil with onion and garlic for five minutes, or cut into a salad.

Dandelion Root Medicinal:

Pull dandelions from the garden, (if you do not use chemicals on your lawn), preferably before the plant begins to flower in the early spring. Wash the roots, slice in half lengthwise, and chop into small pieces. Spread the pieces out in one layer and allow them to dry in a cool, dry, shady place for two to three weeks before using them in teas, infusions, or decoctions.

Dandelion Tea:

Steep 1/4 teaspoon of dandelion leaves in one cup of boiled water for three minutes.

Dandelion Root Tea:

While Dandelion Root Tea is considered very bitter, when it is lightly prepared, the tea is much milder with an earthy-sweet flavor. Simmer 1/4 to 1/2 teaspoon of root in two cups of water for five minutes for a gently sweet lactogenic medicinal.

Dandelion Tincture:

Take one to two milliliters, or 10 to 15 drops, of tincture three times per day.

Dandelion Infusion:

Soak one tablespoon of dandelion roots in three cups of cold water overnight. In the morning, briefly boil the infusion on the stove top and strain. Drink one cup 30 minutes before meals.

Dandelion Decoction:

Gently simmer one tablespoon of finely chopped fresh, dried, or powdered dandelion root in three cups of water for 10 to 15 minutes before drinking.

Combined Dandelion Decoction:

Simmer 1/4 teaspoon each of dandelion root, fenugreek seeds, and marshmallow root in three cups of water for 10 to 15 minutes before drinking.

As a supplement in capsule form, follow the recommended dosages directions listed on the package.

Dill Tea:

Steep one teaspoon of crushed dill seeds in a cup of boiled water for 10 to 15 minutes. Drink three to six cups of tea throughout the day.

Light Dill Tea:

Steep one teaspoon of dill seeds in a cup of boiling water for three minutes. Sweeten to taste. Drink three to six cups of tea throughout the day.

Dill Decoction:

Soak three tablespoons of dill seed in a quart of boiling water overnight. In the morning, gently simmer the mixture on the stove top until half or more of the liquid has evaporated. Drink the decoction throughout the day.

Echinacea Tincture:

As a healing medicinal, take 15-30 drops of tincture three to five times a day for one day, and then reduce the dosage to three times a day until your condition improves.

As a lactogenic, take 15-30 drops of tincture three times a day for up to two weeks.

As a supplement in capsule form, follow the dosage directions listed on the package.

Fennel Tea:

Gently crush one to two teaspoons of fennel seeds, and add one cup of boiling water. Cover the cup and steep for five to 20 minutes. Longer steeping produces a more potent tea. Sweeten to taste.

Light Fennel Tea:

Follow the directions as above, but steep for only one to three minutes for a milder taste and effect.

Fennel Infusion:

Place a handful of fennel seeds in a quart jar and cover with boiling water. Cover the jar tightly and allow to steep for a minimum of four hours before drinking.

Cold Fennel Infusion:

Placed a handful of fennel seeds in a quart of cold water and soak them overnight. The following day, strain the liquid and gently warm it on a stove top before drinking. Cold infusion ensures that none of the herb's volatile, medicinal oil is lost to steam.

The usual recommended dosage of Fennel Teas and Infusions is three cups per day. To increase milk production, take up to six cups a day initially, as necessary, but be sure to observe your reaction to this supplement,. If you experience any side effects, reduce the dosage, or discontinue use, and consider using a different galactagogue.

Fenugreek Tea:

Fenugreek seed can be adjusted to be either mild and delicate or potent and bitter, depending on how many seeds are added to water, and how long they are steeped. Pour eight ounces of boiling water over one to three teaspoons of fenugreek seeds and allow to steep for five to 20 minutes before drinking. Sweeten to taste.

Cold Fenugreek Infusion:

Place one cup of Fenugreek seeds in cold water and soak for several hours or overnight. In the morning, strain off the liquid and refrigerate. Each cup of the infusion can be gently warmed on the stove top before drinking.

Fenugreek Decoction:

Add 1 1/2 teaspoons of slightly crushed fenugreek seeds and one teaspoon of anise to one cup of water and gently simmer on the stove top for 10 minutes. Drink the decoction three times per day.

As a supplement, begin by taking one capsule; gauge your response to the supplement. If you do not have an allergic reaction, take three capsules the following day, dividing the dosage into three equal amounts, taken before meals. Build the dosage slowly, adding one capsule per day, until you have reached the recommended standard daily dose of nine capsules. Continue to monitor your reaction to the capsules carefully. Some women see a good improvement in their milk supply by taking only two capsules per day.

Fenugreek can be taken in conjunction with alfalfa leaf, blessed thistle, marshmallow root, and red clover, and while you can combine one or more of these herbs, it is important to remember that specific combinations will work differently for every woman, so choose a combination that is best for you, and gauge your reaction and response to the combined supplements carefully. Divide the combined lactogenic treatment into three daily doses, taking each one before meals.

The recommended combination dosage is:

Fenugreek: One to three capsules
Alfalfa leaf: One to three capsules
Blessed thistle: One to three capsules
Marshmallow Root:: One to three capsules
Red Clover: One to three capsules

Garlic:

You can chop and sautee fresh garlic cloves in virgin olive oil, adding them to a variety of dishes, to take advantage of the flavor, medicinal, and lactogenic **properties it** provides.

As a supplement in capsule form, take one to three garlic pills per day.

Goat's Rue Tea:

Pour one cup of boiling water over one teaspoon of dried goat's rue. Steep for five to 10 minutes. Sweeten to taste. Drink two to three cups of tea per day.

Goat's Rue Tincture:

Take one to two milliliters, or 10 to 15 drops, of tincture beneath the tongue two to three times per day.

Hops Tea:

Pour one cup of boiling water onto one teaspoon of the dried hops flowers, and steep for 10 to 15 minutes. Take one cup in the late afternoon, evening, or just before bedtime. Because hops is classified as a bitter, it should only be lightly sweetened.

Marshmallow Root Tea:

Pour one cup of cold water over one tablespoon of root powder, and stir frequently while soaking for 30 minutes. Strain, and gently warm the liquid on the stove top before drinking. Sweeten to taste.

Marshmallow Root Decoction:

Per cup of water, add one teaspoonful of the chopped marshmallow root, and simmer on the stove top for 10 to 15 minutes. Drink three cups a day.

As a supplement in capsule form, take up to three capsules, three times per day, in combination with other herbs such as fenugreek, blessed thistle, alfalfa, and red clover.

Nettle Leaf Tea:

Pour a cup of boiled water onto one to two teaspoons of dried nettle leaf, cover the cup, and steep for 10 minutes. Drink three cups a day. To kick-start milk production, double this dosage, and drink up to six cups of tea a day.

Light Nettle Leaf Tea:

Steep one teaspoon of the dried herb for only 1/2 minute in a cup of boiling water. Drink three cups a day. Even this mild tea version has a dark-green color and a rich taste.

Nettle Infusion:

In a quart jar, add one large handful of nettle leaf and cover with boiling water. Cover the jar tightly, and infuse overnight. The next morning, gently warm one cup of the infusion on the stove top, and sweeten before drinking. Drink three cups per day.

Combined Nettle Infusion:

You can combine nettle leaf with other lactogenic herbs,

such as alfalfa, goat's rue, dandelion leaf, red clover, and umbel seeds, and infuse as directed above.

Red Clover Tea:

Pour one cup of boiling water onto one to three teaspoons of the dried red clover flowers, and steep for 10 to 15 minutes. Sweeten to taste. Drink up to three cups of tea per day.

Red Clover Infusion:

Blend several teaspoons of red clover with a variety of other lactogenic herbs, and place them in a quart jar. Cover the herbs with boiling water, and allow them to steep overnight. In the morning, gently warm one cup of infusion on the stove top before drinking. Take three cups per day.

As a supplement, take two to three red clover capsules three times a day, in combination with other lactogenic herbs.

Red Raspberry Leaf Tea:

Pour one cup of boiling water over two teaspoons of dried raspberry leaf and steep for five minutes. Sweeten to taste. Drink two to three cups of tea per day for a maximum of two weeks.

Light Red Raspberry Leaf Tea:

Steep 1/2 teaspoon of dried red raspberry leaves in one cup of boiling water for one to three minutes. Sweeten to taste. Drink up to three cups of light tea for a maximum of two weeks.

Vervain Tea:

Pour one cup of boiling water onto one to three teaspoons of dried verbena and steep for 10 to 15 minutes. Sweeten to taste. Drink three cups of tea per day.

Light Vervain Tea:

Steep1/2 to one teaspoon of dried herb for one to three minutes in a cup of boiled water. Add stevia or other natural sweeteners to taste. Drink three cups of light tea per day.

Umbel Seed Single Tea:

Gently crush two teaspoons of the umbel seed of your choice, and add one cup of boiling water to the herb. Cover the cup and steep for five to 20 minutes. Longer steeping produces a more potent tea. Sweeten to taste.

Umbel Seed Combination Tea:

Gently crush one teaspoon each of the umbel seeds of your choice, and add one cup of boiling water to the herbs. Cover the cup and steep for five to 20 minutes. Longer steeping produces a more potent tea. Sweeten to taste.

Light Umbel Seed Single Tea:

Gently crush one teaspoon of the seed of your choice and cover with boiling water. Steep one to three minutes for a milder taste and effect. Sweeten to taste.

Light Umbel Seed Combination Tea:

Gently crush one teaspoon each of the seeds of your choice and cover with boiling water. Steep one to three minutes for a milder taste and effect. Sweeten to taste.

Umbel Seed Infusions:

In Eastern Europe, umbel seeds, such as anise, given to breastfeeding women to promote milk production, are covered with boiling water and infused for a minimum of four hours before consuming, while in India, the umbel seeds are placed in cold water and soaked overnight. The liquid is strained and gently warmed before drinking. By using this method of infusion, it is believed that none of the volatile, medicinal oil is lost to steam.

Traditional Infusion:

Select a combination of umbel seeds to use in your infusion, and add one cup of each to a pint jar. Cover the seeds with boiling water, filling the jar to the top. Place a lid on the jar and allow to steep for a minimum of four hours before drinking.

Cold Infusion:

Select a combination of umbel seeds to use in your infusion, and add one cup of each to a pint jar. Cover the seeds with cold water, filling the jar to the top. Place a lid on the jar and allow to steep overnight. Once your cold infusion is ready, strain the liquid before drinking.

The recommended dosage of Umbel Seed Tea and Infusions is three cups per day. To increase milk production more quickly, drink up to six cups of tea per day. Gauge your response and reaction to the umbel seeds carefully. If you begin to notice a significant increase in your milk supply, lower your dose back to three cups of tea each day.

Chapter 6
Lactation Tea Recipes

Mama's Milk Anise Herbal Lactation Tea

This hydrating lactation tea is filled with vitamins, minerals, and key nutrients to support the immune system and boost and enrich breast milk supply. Enjoy three to six cups per day, and consider drinking a cup before bed, to encourage morning milk flow.

You will need:

- ❖ 1/2 cup anise seeds
- ❖ 1/2 cup red raspberry leaf
- ❖ 1/4 cup nettle leaf
- ❖ 1/4 cup alfalfa
- ❖ 1/4 cup dandelion leaf
- ❖ 1/4 cup blessed thistle
- ❖ 1 cinnamon stick, crushed
- ❖ A few cloves

To blend your tea:

Combine all herbs, cinnamon, and cloves in a bowl. Store your tea blend in a glass airtight container with a well-fitting lid in a cool, dry, dark place to preserve freshness for up to three months.

To prepare your tea:

Place two teaspoons of blended tea in a cup, and cover with eight ounces of boiling water. Allow to steep for 10 minutes.

Serving suggestions:

Lightly sweeten with honey. Add a dash of cream and lemon for flavor.

Mama's Milk Caraway Herbal Lactation Tea

This hydrating lactation tea is filled with vitamins, minerals, and key nutrients to support the immune system and boost and enrich breast milk supply. Enjoy three to six cups per day, and consider drinking a cup before bed, to encourage morning milk flow.

You will need:

❖ 1/2 cup caraway seeds
❖ 1/2 cup red raspberry leaf
❖ 1/4 cup nettle leaf
❖ 1/4 cup alfalfa
❖ 1/4 cup dandelion leaf
❖ 1/4 cup blessed thistle
❖ 1 cinnamon stick, crushed
❖ A few cloves

To blend your tea:

Combine all herbs, cinnamon, and cloves in a bowl. Store your tea blend in a glass airtight container with a well-fitting lid in a cool, dry, dark place to preserve freshness for up to three months.

To prepare your tea:

Place two teaspoons of blended tea in a cup, and cover with eight ounces of boiling water. Allow to steep for 10 minutes.

Serving suggestions:

Lightly sweeten with honey. Add a dash of cream and lemon for flavor.

Mama's Milk Coriander Herbal Lactation Tea

This hydrating lactation tea is filled with vitamins, minerals, and key nutrients to support the immune system and boost and enrich breast milk supply. Enjoy three to six cups per day, and consider drinking a cup before bed, to encourage morning milk flow.

You will need:

* ❖ 1/2 cup coriander seeds
* ❖ 1/2 cup red raspberry leaf
* ❖ 1/4 cup nettle leaf
* ❖ 1/4 cup alfalfa
* ❖ 1/4 cup dandelion leaf
* ❖ 1/4 cup blessed thistle
* ❖ 1 cinnamon stick, crushed
* ❖ A few cloves

To blend your tea:

Combine all herbs, cinnamon, and cloves in a bowl.

Store your tea blend in an airtight container with a well-fitting lid in a cool dry dark place to preserve freshness.

To prepare your tea:

Place two teaspoons of blended tea in a cup, and cover with eight ounces of boiling water. Allow to steep for 10 minutes.

Serving suggestions:

Lightly sweeten with honey. Add a dash of cream and lemon for flavor.

Mama's Milk Cumin Herbal Lactation Tea

This hydrating lactation tea is filled with vitamins, minerals, and key nutrients to support the immune system and boost and enrich breast milk supply. Enjoy three to six cups per day, and consider drinking a cup before bed, to encourage morning milk flow.

You will need:

- 1/2 cup fennel seeds
- 1/2 cup red raspberry leaf
- 1/4 cup nettle leaf
- 1/4 cup alfalfa
- 1/4 cup dandelion leaf
- 1/4 cup blessed thistle
- 1 cinnamon stick, crushed
- A few cloves

To blend your tea:

Combine all herbs, cinnamon, and cloves in a bowl. Store your tea blend in a glass airtight container with a well-fitting lid in a cool, dry, dark place to preserve freshness for up to three months.

To prepare your tea:

Place two teaspoons of blended tea in a cup, and cover with eight ounces of boiling water. Allow to steep for 10 minutes.

Serving suggestions:

Lightly sweeten with honey. Add a dash of cream and lemon for flavor.

Mama's Milk Dill Herbal Lactation Tea

This hydrating lactation tea is filled with vitamins, minerals, and key nutrients to support the immune system and boost and enrich breast milk supply. Enjoy three to six cups per day, and consider drinking a cup before bed, to encourage morning milk flow.

You will need:

- 1/2 cup dill seeds
- 1/2 cup red raspberry leaf
- 1/4 cup nettle leaf
- 1/4 cup alfalfa
- 1/4 cup dandelion leaf
- 1/4 cup blessed thistle
- 1 cinnamon stick, crushed
- A few cloves

To blend your tea:

Combine all herbs, cinnamon, and cloves in a bowl. Store your tea blend in a glass airtight container with a well-fitting lid in a cool, dry, dark place to preserve freshness for up to three months.

To prepare your tea:

Place two teaspoons of blended tea in a cup, and cover with eight ounces of boiling water. Allow to steep for 10 minutes.

Serving suggestions:

Lightly sweeten with honey. Add a dash of cream and lemon for flavor.

Mama's Milk Fennel Herbal Lactation Tea

This hydrating lactation tea is filled with vitamins, minerals, and key nutrients to support the immune system and boost and enrich breast milk supply. Enjoy three to six cups per day, and consider drinking a cup before bed, to encourage morning milk flow.

You will need:

* 1/2 cup fennel seeds
* 1/2 cup red raspberry leaf
* 1/4 cup nettle leaf
* 1/4 cup alfalfa
* 1/4 cup dandelion leaf
* 1/4 cup blessed thistle
* 1 cinnamon stick, crushed

❖   A few cloves

To blend your tea:

Combine all herbs, cinnamon, and cloves   in a bowl. Store your tea blend in a glass airtight container with a well-fitting lid in a cool, dry, dark place to preserve freshness for up to three months.

To prepare your tea:

Place two teaspoons of blended tea in a cup, and cover with eight ounces of boiling water. Allow to steep for 10 minutes.

Serving suggestions:

Lightly sweeten with honey. Add a dash of cream and lemon for flavor.

Mama's Milk Herbal Iced Lactation Tea

This fabulous drink is a wonderful alternative to traditional hot nursing teas. Using just three key lactogenics, this iced tea is easy to prepare, using a traditional infusion method before chilling.

You will need:

❖   1 tablespoon fennel seeds
❖   1 tablespoon fenugreek seeds
❖   1/2 tablespoon dill seeds
❖   1 gallon of water

To prepare your tea:

Place one gallon of water in a pot, and bring to a boil on the stove top, over medium-high heat. Add the herbs to the boiling water, reduce heat, and simmer for 30 minutes. Remove the pan from the heat and allow the infusion to cool completely.

To store your tea:

Once the infusion has cooled, pour it into individual-sized water bottles with well-fitting caps and store it in the refrigerator for up to 36 hours.

Serving suggestions:

Prior to packaging your tea, you can sweeten the cooled infusion with honey and lemon.

Nursing Power Herbal Lactation Tea

This hydrating lactation tea is filled with 13 powerful vitamin, mineral, and nutrient enriched galactagogues to support the immune system and greatly increase and enrich breast milk supply. Enjoy three to six cups per day, and consider drinking a cup before bed, to encourage morning milk flow. Gauge your body's response to this lactation tea carefully. If you notice a dramatic increase in milk supply, reduce the daily dose to no more than three cups of tea per day.

You will need:
- ❖ 2 teaspoons fenugreek seeds
- ❖ 2 teaspoons fennel seeds
- ❖ 2 teaspoons coriander seeds

- ❖ 2 teaspoons cumin seeds
- ❖ 2 teaspoons cardamom seeds
- ❖ 2 teaspoons nettle leaf
- ❖ 2 teaspoons red raspberry leaf
- ❖ 1 teaspoon dandelion leaf
- ❖ 2 teaspoons alfalfa powder
- ❖ 2 teaspoons oat straw powder
- ❖ 2 teaspoons German chamomile powder
- ❖ 2 teaspoons ginger
- ❖ 2 cinnamon sticks, lightly crushed

To prepare your tea:

Place herbs, seeds, powders, and spices in a pint-sized glass jar and shake gently to blend. Cover the tea blend with boiling water, filling the jar to the top. Cover tightly with a well-fitting lid and allow to steep, for a minimum of one hour. For best results, brew the infusion overnight.

When your infusion is ready, strain the herbs from the liquid, and enjoy this lactation tea throughout the day. Store any left-over tea in the refrigerator for up to 36 hours.

Serving suggestions:

Lightly sweeten with honey. Add lemon for additional flavor.

Blessed Borage Nursing Tea

This lactation tea is filled with vitamins, minerals, and key nutrients to support the immune system, balance the hormones, and boost and enrich breast milk supply. Begin by drinking just one cup of this tea per day. Gauge your body's response to this lactogenic carefully. After a week, if necessary, increase the dosage to two cups of Blessed Borage Tea per day. If you notice a dramatic increase in milk supply, reduce the daily dose once more.

You will need:

- ❖ 1 ounce borage leaves
- ❖ 1 ounce blessed thistle
- ❖ 1 ounce red raspberry leaf
- ❖ 1 ounce fenugreek seeds

To blend your tea:

Combine herbs and fenugreek seeds in a small bowl. Store in a glass airtight container with a well-fitting lid in a cool, dark, dry place to preserve freshness for up to three months.

To prepare your tea:

Place one teaspoon of tea in a cup. Cover with eight ounces of boiling water. Allow to steep for 10 minutes before drinking.

Serving suggestions:

Lightly sweeten with honey. Add a pinch of cinnamon and lemon for additional flavor.

Chamomile Nursing Tea

This soothing lactation tea is filled with vitamins, minerals, and key nutrients to support the immune system, boost and enrich breast milk supply, and aid with the let down reflex. Enjoy three to six cups of tea per day, and consider having a cup before bed to improve sleep and morning milk flow.

You will need:

* ❖ 1/2 cup red raspberry leaf
* ❖ 1/2 cup nettle leaf
* ❖ 1/4 cup fenugreek seeds
* ❖ 1/4 cup fennel seeds
* ❖ 1/4 cup alfalfa leaf
* ❖ 1/4 cup dandelion leaf
* ❖ 1/4 cup chamomile flowers

To blend your tea:

Combine herbs, seeds, and flowers in a small bowl. Store your blend in a glass airtight container with a well-fitting lid in a cool, dark, dry place to preserve freshness for up to three months.

To prepare one cup of tea:

Add two cups of water to a saucepan and bring to a boil on the stove top over medium-high heat. Add one tablespoon of tea, reduce heat, and simmer for 15 minutes. Strain before drinking.

To prepare one gallon of tea:

In a large pot on the stove top, bring one gallon of water to a boil over medium-high heat. Add 1/2 cup tea blend, reduce heat, and simmer for 15 minutes. Strain. Place tea in a pitcher and refrigerate tea for up to 36 hours.

Chilled tea can be re-warmed on the stove top by the cup.

Serving suggestions:

Lightly sweeten with honey. Add a pinch of cinnamon, lemon, and a dash of cream for additional flavor.

Lemon Verbena Nursing Tea

This uplifting lactation tea is filled with vitamins, minerals, and key nutrients to support the immune system, boost and enrich breast milk supply, and aid with the let down reflex. Enjoy three cups of tea per day, and consider having a cup before bed to improve sleep and morning milk flow.

You will need:

- ❖ 1/2 cup nettle leaf
- ❖ 1/2 cup red raspberry leaf
- ❖ 1/2 cup lemon verbena
- ❖ 1/4 cup fenugreek seeds
- ❖ 1/4 cup fennel seeds
- ❖ 1/4 cup blessed thistle

To prepare your blend:

Combine all herbs and seeds in a small bowl. Store the blend in a glass airtight container with a well-fitting lid in a cool, dry, dark place to preserve freshness for up to three months.

To prepare one cup of tea:

Place one teaspoon of tea blend in a cup and cover with eight ounces of boiling water. Steep for five minutes before drinking.

To prepare a pot of tea:

Use one teaspoon of tea to every cup of boiling water. Allow the herbs to steep for 10 minutes before serving.

Serving suggestions:

Lightly sweeten with honey. Add a dash of cream for additional flavor.

Chapter 7
The Garden Bounty:
A Nutritive Summary

Years ago, my mother-in-law told me the story of her childhood growing up in the mountains of West Virginia when, every spring and summer, she and her sisters would forage for plants and berries so their family could eat. Times were very rough and money was scarce, but, somehow, her mother managed to feed eight hungry children, sometimes on nothing more than dandelion greens and clover and wild raspberries that grew so plentifully in the Appalachians. This experience taught my mother-in-law that viable food sources abound, and gave her a deep appreciation of nature and gardening.

Herbs truly are one of nature's greatest gifts to us, and not only are the lactogenic variety good for our breast milk supply, they can be good for our *bodies*, too, boosting the immune system and fortifying us with important vitamins, minerals, and nutrients. Here are just some of the many benefits you'll find in the galactagogues listed in this guide.

Alfalfa:

Known as the "father of all foods", alfalfa is rich in vitamins K and C and chlorophyll, and is used as an ingredient in many multivitamins because it helps to alleviate fluid retention and swelling, promotes a healthy urinary and digestive tract, and cleanses the blood as it rebuilds vitality and boosts breast milk supply.

Blessed Thistle:

This is one of the best galactagogues for increasing and enriching breast milk supply, and is a wonderful way to restore the nursing woman's vitality.

Borage:

This herb is an excellent source of Vitamins C and A, iron, calcium, potassium, copper, zinc, magnesium, and essential fatty acids.

Chamomile:

This calming and soothing herb promotes relaxation and restful sleep for Mom *and* baby, and aids in the let down reflex.

Dandelion Leaf:

The benefits of this herb are quite extensive. Not only is it a wonderful source of fiber and rich in vitamins A, C, D, and B, iron, magnesium, zinc, potassium, manganese, copper, choline, calcium, boron, and silicon, it is a natural diuretic that alleviates fluid retention.

Echinacea:

A restorative that cleanses and purifies, echinacea helps to support the immune system.

Fenugreek:

Fenugreek has been used for centuries as a natural breast enhancer, enlarger, and galactagogue that not only dramatically increases milk production and supply, but also improves the overall health and beauty of the breasts. Along with vitamin C and potassium, fenugreek also contains diosgenin, which is said to give this lactogenic its milk-making magic.

Nettle Leaf:

High in vitamin C, calcium, iron, and potassium, nettle leaf cleanses the body, improves circulation, and promotes kidney function. Not only does it increase the flow of breast milk, nettle is also believed to help in the prevention and treatment of some skin diseases, such as eczema and psoriasis.

Red Raspberry Leaf:

A soothing herb rich in calcium, vitamin C, magnesium, and potassium, red raspberry leaf is beneficial to the female reproductive system and promotes hormone health as it enriches breast milk supply.

Umbel Seeds:

This "family" includes anise, caraway, coriander, cumin, dill, and fennel, and each seed contains a variety of nutritive properties. As antioxidants that purify the blood, umbel seeds are also known for their anti-inflammatory and anti-viral properties, which help to support the immune system. They are also rich sources of B-complex vitamins, fiber, calcium, manganese, iron, niacin, riboflavin, thiamin, copper, potassium, zinc, magnesium, folate, vitamin C, and essential fatty acids, all which play key roles in promoting increased lactation and enriching breast milk. Not only does fennel stimulate milk production, it improves digestion, and is believed to alleviate tummy upsets and colic in infants as it passes through the breast milk.

Vervain (Lemon Verbena):

This hydrating and uplifting herb helps to alleviate stress and depression as it supports the immune system and aids in successful let down.

Reference Guide

Measurement Conversions

Cup	C or c
Gallon	gal
Gram	g
Liter	l
Milligram	mg
Milliliters	mL or ml
Ounce	oz.
Pint	pt.
Pound	lb.
Quart	qt.
Tablespoon	T. or tbsp.
Teaspoon	Tsp. or t.

Dried Herbs Conversion

Roots	1 ounce is	1 cup or	30 grams
Leaves	1 ounce is	1 cup or	30 grams
Flowers	1 ounce is	1 cup or	30 grams
Seeds	1 ounce is	1 cup or	30 grams

Water Conversion

2 cups is equal to	1 pint
4 cups is equal to	1 quart
16 cups is equal to	1 gallon
1 pint is equal to	500 mL
2 pints is equal to	1 quart
8 pints is equal to	1 gallon
1 quart is equal to	1 liter
4 quarts is equal to	1 gallon
1,000 mL is equal to	1 liter

Infusion Guide
(Using dried herbs)

Roots	1 ounce or 1 cup or 30 grams	1 pint or 500 mL of water	Infuse for a minimum of 8 hours
Leaves	1 ounce or 1 cup or 30 grams	1 quart or 1 liter of water	Infuse for a minimum of 4 hours
Flowers	1 ounce or 1 cup or 30 grams	1 quart or 1 liter of water	Infuse for a minimum of 2 hours
Seeds	1 ounce or 1 cup or 30 grams	1 pint or 500 mL of water	Infuse for a minimum of 30 minutes

Tincture Drops to Milliliters

10 drops of tincture is approximately	1 mL
15 drops of tincture is approximately	2 mL
20 drops of tincture is approximately	3 mL
25 drops of tincture is approximately	4 mL
30 drops of tincture is approximately	5 mL

Afterword and Acknowledgments

I hope you enjoyed *A Fountain of Gardens*, which can be used alone, or alongside my book, *The Art of Lactation,* which explores timeless, tried-and-true lactation techniques used successfully throughout the years by women who dream of creating non-maternal breast milk and those who hope to increase, support, and maintain an established milk supply. Writing these books has been a true pleasure and a blessing in my life. I hope they have somehow blessed you, too.

I would like to extend my gratitude and heartfelt thanks to Holly, Elaine, Christy, and Rebecca, the team of nurses, lactation consultants, and herbalists who worked alongside me during the writing of this book, for their valuable advice, assistance, and time.

May your fountains overflow!

With warm regards,

The Loving Milk Maid

About the Author

Known to readers around the world as the Loving Milk Maid, or simply LMM, blogger and freelance writer Jennifer Elisabeth Maiden first gained recognition with the launch of her original blog, "Bountiful Fruits: A Loving ANR Journey", and now runs the successful website Bountiful Fruits and writes for the natural lifestyle blog, Vintage Rose. Her work has now reached readers throughout the United States and in 28 countries. Ms. Maiden resides in Ohio with her family where she is currently working on her debut fiction novella, *The Flames of Autumn.*